Walk With Me

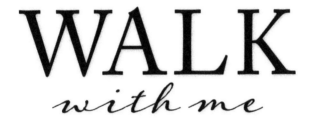

WALK
with me

Adrienne Rea

XULON PRESS

Xulon Press
2301 Lucien Way #415
Maitland, FL 32751
407.339.4217
www.xulonpress.com

© 2019 by Adrienne Rea

Unless otherwise indicated, Scripture quotations taken
from the Holy Bible, New International Version (NIV).
Copyright © 1973, 1978, 1984, 2011 by Biblica, Inc.™.
Used by permission. All rights reserved.

Printed in the United States of America.

ISBN-13: 978-1-54566-796-5

Against all odds

One woman's journey from illness to full health and another woman coming alongside to be a part of the miracle journey. A journey totally planned by our Lord Jesus. From ten years of being chained to a dialysis machine for three nights a week, four hours at a time, to being set free from all of this and being given newness of life, hope for a future away from hospitals. This book wants to bring inspiration and joy to others out there who are pulled down by illness. Whatever your plight is right now, remember that we serve a mighty God and he's still performing miracles today.

Adriennes story (donor)

*I*t is exactly 23 weeks to the day since surgery to transplant my kidney into Lorraine. As I sit outside in the sunshine of this beautiful warm spring day, I can't help but go over in my mind all the events that took place on November 7th 2014. It seems a life time ago now but as I begin to reflect, it stirs up a lot of emotions and takes me right back. With surgery having taken place early on the Friday morning that whole day passed by in a bit of a blur.

I can recall the previous night fasting, then wakening up early to pre surgical procedures, final blood tests and forms to be signed. Then a chance to speak briefly to Lorraine before my bed was wheeled out heading towards a large lift which took me to a lower floor.

I was extremely calm with no doubts, or concerns about the procedure. I knew you see that this day had been months in the planning by doctors, but a lifetime of planning by our creator God.

I was secure in that knowledge most of all. You see Lorraine and I had watched as our great God had opened doors and performed miracles to get us to this day and this moment, so the end of the story could only be glorious for both of us.

I invite you now to journey with me as I show you the amazing plan of God in what seemed like an impossible task, to give Lorraine the opportunity to live an abundant life, free from that illness which had blighted most of her life, having been born with polycystic kidney disease. We know our God could have sorted it all out with one touch, yet instead he chose to do the miracle in a different way and involving myself. That dear readers is a miracle in itself, to get me to a place where I would agree to undergo surgery, to have one of my kidneys transplanted into my friend, and even more so as we weren't even a good match for any safe transplant procedure. Please journey with me and meet our lovely Lord and Saviour Jesus Christ.

Life is a production
God is the chief producer
All have leading roles to play.

God doesn't look for outer beauty but beauty from within, put there by Himself from the rebirth. Inner strength, patience, kindness, gentleness, peace, love and a willingness to take part, whatever the character role entails. He spends a lifetime preparing you for your moment, shaping you with every trial, changing you through life's circumstances, moulding you like the potter to the clay. Then when he knows you are ready, he begins the audition asking, "Will you?". He already knows the ending; he knows it's going to be a great production, much talked about, but you don't yet understand. You simply must follow his lead. If he knows that you are the most suitable person to be his leading character then how can you say no ?

> "And I know the plans I have for you declares the Lord, plans to prosper you and not harm you, plans to give you hope and a future."
>
> Jeremiah ch29.v11

Seventeen years ago one Sunday morning, my husband Irvine and I strapped the children into the car and headed out of the house to go to church. Church for us at that time was the local Presbyterian in Larne town centre. The four children were used to the Sunday morning routine, although it was never without a drama. Warren and Jaclyn being the older two would come rather reluctantly provided they could wear whatever they chose to. Jaclyn being the only girl would make sure that was a football top and tracksuit bottoms. Just getting them all into the car and with minutes

3

before the start of the service was what we had come to expect. The younger two Shane and Mark had been afforded some time over their outfits and generally looked cute. Shane was always smiling and Mark sucked his thumb and loved his hair spiked. This particular Sunday we decided at the last minute to turn left instead of right and head down to the local country church of Cairncastle, by way of a change. In that decision, Gods plan for the next part of my life was taking shape and I didn't know it. I was driving right into the centre of God's will.

Unbeknown to me, on that same Sunday Lorraine and William Harper were sitting upstairs at Cairncastle Church. Apparently they watched us from the upstairs balcony as we were escorted to the front row seats, being late of course! We probably did cause a bit of a stir in that little village community church, where little changes and everybody knows each other. Lorraine told me years later that when she saw us that morning she just knew that I would become a very good friend. What discernment!

Very often as Christians we look for a purpose and a plan in our life according to Gods will. Many times I had been faced with that very thought. Am I living out the purpose God has for me? Is there something God wants me to do in the future and if so, does where I am today line up with that plan?

In my personal experience with getting to know Lorraine, I can say that I had no idea that God wanted me to undergo surgery and to be used by him in this role by God. That is, not until six months before it happened.

It's only on looking back over the last seventeen years, I realise that God had called me and was positioning me in such a way that when the phone call came, I was able to say yes immediately. He had prepared my health, my new home and my work status so that nothing would prevent this from taking place. As a family we had unwittingly been making big life decisions without any knowledge of God being in the centre of all those. Yes we certainly asked for his guidance but never ever knowing the bigger picture. When it was all over and I reflected on all that it blew me away.

For example, the way in which we ended up buying property out at Cairncastle, near to Lorraine and William had Gods plan stamped all over it. We had joined Cairncastle Church after that first Sunday and much later found a property being built nearby. To us a dream to live in the country with our children was being fulfilled, however to God he was moving us right over next to Lorraine's home, so that our friendship would deepen and his plan and purpose would move a step closer to fulfilment.

Adrienne's background

When a young child first finds those beautiful shoes belonging to mum she just has to try them on. Tiny toes slide into high heels. She clip clips around the floor for a few moments pretending to be mummy-wobbly at first then eventually mastering the steps. At last, she must take them off, come back to herself. She isn't fully grown yet. One day she will walk in her own high heels and they will fit just perfectly.

My teaching career felt exactly like that child. I was in a career, however it felt like it was someone else's. I was wobbly, unsure and fell many times. I mastered it for a number of years, eighteen to be exact but it wasn't my calling and finally in 2005, I took off the career shoes and laid them down. I needed to find my own that fitted just perfectly. You see our God had put gifts and talents inside of me and they still had to be found. He had a purpose and a plan for my life, not yet fulfilled. Once more I was moving into his will. This new season in my life brought less stress, more time with my own growing family and especially time to get to know more of God and his word. I discovered I had a real love for creativity and began to try all sorts of new skills. At this most precious time away for full time work I learnt more about myself than ever before. I believe God allowed this time so I could establish a closer relationship with him, for what lay ahead.

Lorraine's story

*L*orraine was born on 9th September 1963 and it was later discovered that she had inherited polycystic kidney disease, just like her mum. Her mum passed away when Lorraine was just thirteen years old and despite this early loss Lorraine coped as well as could be expected.She grew up in a farming community and now being looked after by her father and an aunt. All this made her strong in character, a real fighter.

When I met Lorraine in 2000, she was vibrant. We hit it off immediately despite being worlds apart in our life styles. While she spent a lot of time helping her father on the farm, I was more a town girl, interested in fashions and crafts. Our common ground was our love of the Saviour and our pursuit to know him more. As our friendship grew we attended weekly bible study together. Although friends at our local church would sometimes mention Lorraine's poor health and her need of a transplant, this never really impacted me owing to the fact that Lorraine herself never mentioned her own personal difficulties and always appeared very bright and happy. It was only in 2012 when Lorraine took an infection called peritonitis that I saw firsthand how ill she really was.She had to be admitted to hospital and made it just in time. She was seriously ill for many days. I visited her along with her husband William one evening and saw how poorly she was. This was a wakeup call to me about kidney disease and the potential threat which hung over Lorraine's life.

When you sit in a doctors surgery and you are presented with a 2% chance of ever receiving a kidney match, the odds are greatly stacked against you. When you are then told that the most recent live donor to come forward to be tested doesn't match your tissue type, it doesn't get much worse. When all the scientific evidence would suggest that years of having kidney dialysis could poten- tially have caused a lot of calcification to build up in your veins, making surgery for transplant pretty tricky indeed, you can imagine just how hopeless Lorraine's situation looked.

So when a consultant at the City Hospital Belfast pointed her finger directly at Lorraine one day, early in February 2014 and said," Lorraine this has to be your year for a kidney" little did this lady know she was actually speaking prophetically out over the situation. Thankfully those words lingered with Lorraine and as she repeated them to herself she began to get hopeful.

Adriennes story (continued)

*O*ften I walked my dog Jack around the Sallagh fields. This had a dual purpose, exercise for both of us and a time to communicate in prayer to the Almighty God. One such day early Summer 2012 I walked a much different way, for I was carrying a burden to the Lord. I had seen my friend so ill, near to death and I cried out to God. I was mixed up emotionally-angry, impatient for an answer, despairing for no answer and frustrated. My heart was breaking for my friend. It felt like she was imprisoned somewhere. Life's circumstances had her in chains and only my God could intervene. I've heard it said that God wants us to be truthful with him in prayer, to pour out our heart to him, to cry tears to him and so I did all that, on that particular walk. Why God, had no other relatives come forward by now to be tested as possible donors? How difficult is it really just to get a blood test done?

That day as I opened up my heart in total despair to him I suddenly heard a voice from inside me saying, 'What about you?' I stopped. That couldn't have come from my own conscience. Not in my wildest dreams would I ever have considered that. I considered the question. With the flight of my imagination, my mind went off to a hospital scene, me having surgery, Lorraine getting my kidney, family all coming to visit, a great result. Was God asking me to take on this role, a living donor for Lorraine? The thought just wouldn't leave me.

Isn't that our God? So often when we call out to him looking for an answer to a problem, he looks right back at you smiling because he knows you are the solution, and he's actually waiting upon you. Could that be a thought for you the reader to linger upon in your own life, whatever your situation? That day I decided to give a blood sample.

I phoned Lorraine to let her know of my decision. For that first year only Lorraine and William knew about it. I had made up my mind that until we got any positive answer, my own family didn't need to know. I suppose upon reflection this was protection for them. Also playing in my mind was Lorraine's situation being so rare that possibly God was in fact only testing me to see if I was willing and after that there would be nothing further! This was me picturing Abraham placing Isaac upon the sacrificial alter and God would say to me this was all a test of obedience to hearing his voice and nothing more would be required of me. With all this going through my head, I proceeded.

Lorraine was over the moon when she heard. I have often reflected back to that moment and I will probably never fully understand what hope, what joy must come upon a person to hear of a possibility that their life can be turned around. She gave me the contact number for the team up at the City hospital and I took it from there.

To say that the team of doctors I met up there were amazing, doesn't do them justice at all. Each one of them was determined, caring, professional and had just one agenda with Lorraine's situation, to get her a successful kidney transplant, with the best possible chance of success.

The first series of blood tests were all done in Autumn of 2012 in the same afternoon. At that first meeting with me doctor Courtney, she asked me honestly why I wanted to come forward. That was my opportunity to bring God into the conversation and I did. I told her how Lorraine and I shared a common faith in God and I told her how I felt it had been His prompting to come forward for testing. It was only much later on I was to discover that I was in fact speaking to a Christian doctor and she had been praying into Lorraine and many other patients' impossible situations, asking God for his help and intervention.

Weeks passed, Autumn turning to Winter in 2012, until finally a letter came in from the hospital, explaining that although our blood groups matched, our tissue type didn't, so surgery was impossible. I had mixed emotions that morning. Total disappointment for Lorraine who would have received the same letter, yet to be honest, a relief that surgery wasn't being asked of me. I must have been right. God was just looking for my willingness and nothing more. Someone else would likely be used instead and I thanked God for his answer. Life could move forward and my family need never know I had gone to be tested. Lorraine's heart response however must have been totally different! I will never know what disappointment feels like for someone like her right at that moment. To have all hope taken away again, and thoughts of the endless routine on dialysis continuing indefinitely must have been heartbreaking. But remember I have already said that she is a fighter! She has the greatest ability to pick herself up, brush off the disappointment and get on with life as best as she can.

I put the letter away, put surgery totally out of my mind and thanked the Lord for the experience, for the opportunity to share in what could have been a great journey of healing. It also allowed me to get a glimpse into Lorraine's hospital regime and to meet some terrific doctors. To me it had ended as quickly as it had begun. To the Lord however, it had moved a step closer to fulfilment of his plan for Lorraine. My name, my personal details and blood group were all now on file, stored in records. This was not the end at all, but just the beginning. We serve a mighty God !

When a seed is dropped into the soil, it is invisible to the human eye. It is still there to those who tend and water it. One day a new flower will bud, peeping its head up through the soil. Until that day, it remains in the dark.however it's in that place of being hidden that the miracle is taking place. God works out miracles in the secret places, in troubled areas of our lives he says,"Don't despair, I' m at work, wait and see. To God a 'no ' from man can be turned into a ' yes' from Him. We must believe when man says something is impossible, God can make it possible. God can make a way when there is no way.

So as doctors saw Lorraine's antibodies and compared them to 'Trojan horses',rejecting anything that would come into Lorraine's body our great God was actually preparing to open a door to surgery. A door which said 'No entry, antibodies at work! 'God was saying '

"With me all things are possible".

In Luke's gospel ch. 17 v11-19 Jesus met ten lepers who said " Jesus, Master have mercy on us ". Jesus asked them to go show themselves to the priests. And so it was as they went they were cleansed. The lepers had to do something in order to be healed. They obeyed the Masters command and as they began to make their way to the priests, I can just picture their bodies being healed. This healing miracle helped me to see that not every miracle was performed by a touch, but often by a process taking place. Many times as I think about the timing of Lorraine's surgery I am so aware of the miracle of processing, things being put into place at just the right time in order for Lorraine to receive her full healing.

One of those things was a piece of equipment called a Plasma Exchange Machine. In 2014 Guys hospital in London began using this machine on kidney diseased patients leading up to surgery. The machine removed the patients' antibodies and stripped down their immune system. Following this, a new kidney from a donor who wasn't a match, could be inserted and after surgery the immune system was slowly built back up again, and monitored over time to make sure no rejection would occur. It was just in infancy at Guys when Lorraine and I received a phone call in February 2014,to discuss the possibility of surgery in London.

It's **2014**.Two years have passed since I received my letter saying no to surgery being possible. Lorraine had continued on dialysis, with a machine now set up at her home. She was on the machine three times a week, for four hours at a time. Many who came to visit the home wouldn't feel like going down to her bedroom during the treatment, as the noise of the machine made some people uncomfortable and the blood flowing through it put a lot of people off. It was often a lonely sit, as Lorraine wasn't a great television fan. For William and daughter Louise it was a chain upon their lives also. They had to be nearby in case the machine should malfunction or maybe take too much fluid away, leaving Lorraine unwell and in some instances unconscious. They were also a great help at putting the needle into Lorraine's arm to start the whole process. To all who knew Lorraine at this season of her life, it was most evident that she was gravely ill. She couldn't take any breaks away, so holidays were out of the question. She continued to work three days a week and also looked after her dads farmhouse as well as her own. Her faith in Christ kept her believing that God would indeed make a way. She often could be heard thanking the Lord daily for his every provision.

In early February**2014**we were both invited up to Belfast City hospital to speak with Dr. Courtney, the main doctor in charge of Lorraine's case. She explained to us both about the plasma exchange machine. A lot of it was a blur to me, if I'm honest. From yesterday just being an ordinary day, to now seated in this office and being told basically that surgery could be a possibility, I'm in a daze! Can this actually be possible? We would both be invited to fly to London. Lorraine would have a number of sessions on the machine, to prepare her body for surgery, stripping back her immune system, as I have explained. I would be in the hospital for approximately two weeks after surgery and Lorraine's could expect to there for a month. A lot of information was given to us both that day. With it still in its infancy, there weren't a lot of success stories to talk about yet, but Dr Courtney was allowing Lorraine time to think hard about this and not rush into any quick decision.

For me, although it came as a shock that we were back around to the distinct possibility of surgery, for us to have arrived here for a second time, I immediately sensed God has to be in this. As I further reflected upon that and prayed about it I knew my mind was in a different place now and I really began to get stirred up with an excitement of what God was doing. I made it a priority to speak to my family members about the possibility of becoming a live donor for Lorraine. It was certainly a lot for them to take in and many questions were asked by my teenagers. My parents are still alive and so I next told them all about it. Everyone took it very well. They could see my faith in God was uppermost, leading me to make the decision. If God was opening this door, then I was prepared to walk through. I prayed a lot at that time into the whole situation asking for guidance and trusting him for a great healing for the both of us.

As it turned out, after much consideration, Lorraine decided against going to London for the surgery. Two major reasons stopped her. One was the infancy of such a technique and so few success or failure figures to go on. She would have preferred to be having surgery based upon greater success rate since she was so ill at this time.The second reason concerned the distance from home.

To travel to London and be away from family and for a month possibly longer was a deep concern for Lorraine. She is a home girl at heart and to be away from loved ones for so long could affect her recovery physically and emotionally. The Doctor fully understood when after a number of weeks, Lorraine declined the idea completely. Dr Courtney who herself had known Lorraine for years was totally in agreement with her decision. She knew as a professional, that if the patient was in any way unsettled or anxious the whole procedure have less likelihood success.

Therefore the whole plan which was being set up in my head, was no longer going to take place after all. There had been such a shift from that first 'no ' to now suddenly a real possibility. I had such a peace that God was in it. So when Lorraine gave me her decision, I was slightly disappointed. The only thing that now had changed was that my family knew my intention. That was all God must have wanted at that time. This was moving along steadily in God's eyes. I had become very willing to give my kidney and become a live donor. The plasma exchange machine has come into place, albeit in London. A tapestry was being weaved and we aren't yet aware of the pattern emerging. Only God could see the finished work. He alone chooses the colours and the landscape. For a while all we can see is the mess underneath. We must simply trust him that the finished work will look amazing.

A beautiful sunny July morning in the Summer of 2014 I had started the day outside with breakfast. My bible was nearby and I was praying with my eyes open enjoying all the scenery of the countryside around me. The noise of the telephone interrupted my solitude. I took the call which was from the City hospital. The secretary at the other end of the phone couldn't give me a lot of explanation, but apparently I was to attend a meeting at the hospital with Lorraine. We were to meet Dr. Courtney and discuss the possibility of surgery! She did say something about the plasma exchange machine arriving into Belfast with a team of experts who would train staff in Belfast how to use it!

My heart leapt! I saw God in that moment because, just as I had been speaking to him that morning, into the silence had come this call. It had to be God! I began to praise Him, excitement arising within me. My head was putting all the facts together very quickly. I was now standing before an open door and the master was saying, "Walk through. I am ahead of you. I will make the path straight". There was such a peace because of the situation of the phone call coming right at that moment. I just knew the time had arrived for me to take his hand and walk with him, and I was in place of readiness.

It turned out that Lorraine had also received a call. She too was very excited and seemed like myself to understand 2014 was indeed going to be the year for receiving a kidney after all.

From February to July in that year the machine had such a success rate leaving the surgeons to believe it could be of benefit in Belfast. The machine was coming to Belfast and a trained team along with it. The long term implications for kidney surgery here in Belfast would be tremendous, especially for patients like Lorraine who had little chance of ever being matched.

Many meetings took place in the coming months and I don't need to go into every detail. One thing became very clear. I began to see God more and more.

One such encounter came when I met Doctor Courtney to hear all about the machine and talk about Lorraine's antibodies. She produced a chart that day to show me how strong Lorraine's antibodies were behaving. This chart covered the last year. She called the particularly strong antibodies Trojan horses. As soon as my kidney would be put into Lorraine's body these antibodies would rise up to attack and cause rejection, thus surgery would fail. On the chart Lorraine's antibodies had for a long period of time been sitting at eighty to ninety percent in strength. The aim of the machine was to take out all these antibodies, so that transplant could take place. Then slowly reintroduce them after surgery at a very gentle rate so to avoid rejection. It was when Doctor Courtney showed me Lorraine's most recent chart with her antibody strength recorded that I began to see God. No explanation could be given as to why, but those old trojan horses had weakened in strength to fifty percent, allowing a window of opportunity for surgery to take place quite soon. So for no apparent reason and without the use of the machine which was all set to take out those antibodies, they had reduced in strength themselves! God was speaking right at that moment to me, saying, "look at this, do you see my hand at work?". I came out of that meeting knowing that God had spoken again. My peace continued. Lorraine and I were in full agreement that with every meeting, we would fully trust God to open doors or close them. We were trusting him fully with every step.

At another meeting, I shared my faith with the doctor, and told how Lorraine and I were trusting God with it all. Her reply astounded me. It turned out that a group of top surgeons met regularly for prayer for their patients. They had been praying for an opening to come, to be able to help patients who had little chance of ever getting a donor match They could see prayers were being answered. This excited me greatly. To know that the doctors had this set up and were inviting God into their work, confirmed even more that God was walking with us. Lorraine and I took great encouragement from all this knowledge. We were no longer just a couple praying together but now part of a larger prayer team all asking God for a miracle.

I had one full day of tests to be carried out. I was to have every type of check up done from head to toe to make sure I was healthy enough to be a live donor. Most of all my kidney function needed to be assessed to make sure each kidney was working fifty/ fifty. Scans of every description were to be performed. When I got the date confirmed, I rang

Lorraine to tell her and with great joy she told me that the 9 th September, the day of the tests, was her birthday! What a beautiful God we have. He chose that date out of the whole calendar by way of confirming to us that he was in charge and all would be well. What a fantastic birthday gift to be able to phone Lorraine that evening and tell her the results were all looking good and surgery was going ahead. That brought tears of joy.

John ch.10v 27 My sheep hear my voice and I know them and they follow me.

To know that every door being opened was being done so by God gave Lorraine and I such security. We would meet almost every day to walk our dogs, in all sorts of weather and during the period of September through to November we had such a buzz of anticipation as we discussed all that had already happened and prepared for more meetings to come. We laughed together over one meeting in particular that we both had to attend. It was slightly more formal but necessary. We were individually called before a lady to be questioned about our friendship. It was a means to establish how long we had known each other and check that I wasn't in fact receiving large amounts of money for my kidney. We were to come to the meeting and bring a photograph of us together from years ago, thus proving our friendship. The only one time we had taken photographs of each other was during a weekend trip away to Edinburgh. What we didn't realise was that we had none taken together! We laughed at that and the lady totally understood and quickly established that we had been friends since that first church encounter. Lorraine had an important scan to be carried out to make sure that her veins down her legs were capable of coping with a transplant as the kidney was going in at the lower part of her stomach. The doctors were concerned that with a patient on dialysis for so long she could have signs of calcification in her veins, making surgery very difficult. At that time of scan, as the doctors fussed around and got quite excited by the results, Lorraine got anxious to know what was wrong. They quickly reassured her it was nothing, rather the opposite. There was not a sign of any calcification whatsoever! Another check on her heart brought further astonishment because again all looked amazing. To us this was further pushing of doors, more reassurance from our great God. We continued moving forward right up to the week of surgery and that week arrived in November.

Lorraine and I had both reached a place with our faith in God where we felt that He was leading us towards a successful outcome- anything other than this would have been very disappointing. We both met individually with Doctors who spoke truthfully about the implications to us both if surgery wasn't a success. To Lorraine it could mean death. To me it could be a possibility of Lorraine's body rejecting my kidney and me being left with only one kidney and the whole thing a failure. Yet with all the negatives being put in front of us we were steely determined to continue because we had seen God move mightily and we were determined to give him the glory in the outcome.

So the date for surgery was my decision. I picked early November, simply because I knew Lorraine had been told 2014 was her year so I didn't want January 2015. Also my birthday was at the end of November so I thought it would be nice to be home and recovering well by then. The 7 th November was the set date and the plasma machine was booked to arrive in preparation for that date.

We will never know the time and training required by the staff as they got to grips with that machine. However by the first week of November they were all ready for Lorraine to come in and have her immune system stripped away in preparation for surgery.

A doctor explained to her that the whole procedure could leave her dizzy, feeling sick and most likely unable to do much. For two days of that week the treatment began. At no time did Lorraine ever feel ill and she was able to travel home each evening and have a good rest in her own home. We really shouldn't have been surprised! This meant that in the day prior to surgery we could both travel up together, which was very special.

The Thursday morning as I sat preparing to leave, watching the clock, I hadn't a nerve. I d already said goodbye to each family member. Every reassurance was given to them that I was going to be great and would see them soon. I believe they saw my faith in the days leading up to departure by my calmness around the home.

So the final door to go through awaited. I sat to do my morning prayers and read scripture. I sought God in every passage, asking him to give me something personal just between him and myself. He led me to read John ch 10 v 27-28. My sheep hear my voice and I know them and they follow me. Twice in different books I picked up that morning I read that scripture. He hand-picked it for my reassurance. I knew that. What peace came from those words. I knew clearly that I had heard his voice all those years back in the lane.The journey Lorraine and I had been on together had been prepared before we came into existence. With faith and hope for what lay ahead I travelled to pick up Lorraine. As she said her goodbyes to William, I could hear her say to her beloved dog Madge, "see you in a week. " Faith being spoken aloud brings results. We walk by faith and not by sight.

Most of the preparation for surgery passed quickly and in a flurry of activity. So much paper work, identification checks, birth date asked over and over! In all the busyness of the hospital ward there was a calmness around me which never left. My bed was right by the window on the top floor of the city hospital. The views were spectacular. Doctors came and went, menus were passed around for next day to tick. My special consultant was called Elaine, who just happened to be a relative of my husbands. Didn't I mention what a God we have, to assign someone to me who already knew family and could chat in a relaxed manner to me. What a fantastic difference this made. As well as this Doctor Courtney was such a professional and also so able to speak to everyone at their own level. She had such a godly presence when she spoke. I know she was hand picked by God for the task and I thank Him for her.

Lorraine was assigned a private room, but we were close by and I was able to see her most of that day. In the evening our husbands visited us and it was all relaxed and good fun. All final bloods had been checked and we were good to go in the morning. God gave us both a good nights rest and Friday morning came with a rush of activity around my bed. My surgery was first thing and I was leaving the ward near 7:30 am. Lorraine and I had a hug and a prayer. The big moment had arrived.

I picture this part in slow motion even today as I recall it. The large lift that opened to allow my bed to be wheeled inside. The long wide corridors that I was wheeled through with strangers looking on. All so surreal yet calmness within me. Everything prepared by God for this moment. A letting go and trusting God. Wheeled then into an area to receive the injection before sleep. One final stranger reassuring me that the needle going into my arm wouldn't hurt too badly. One final prayer.....keep me Lord under the shelter of your wings.

The rest of that day came and went with little recollection. I woke briefly in recovery, then was wheeled back to the ward. Lorraine was already away into surgery which was to last into the evening. Irvine came to visit and I remember being sick with the first food. Someone came to inform me that Lorraine was out and it was all over and looked good so far. Then more sleep....

The next day was probably the worst for me. Anyone who has had the surgery can share and agree with me, that your body lets you know you have had major surgery. A catheter was still in place and pain relief was taking the edge of the pain but my body ached, there was no doubt. The nurses were insisting that I needed to get out of bed and sit for a while but my body was having second thoughts. Then there were the surgical stockings! What a delight. They were to prevent clotting while lying in bed. I wasn't amused by their look at all. I was given a plastic implement to blow into. This was to improve my breathing which had become quite shallow after surgery. That became like a new toy to be played with for the next few days. When I did begin to move around, the air which had been pumped into my body to remove the kidney, was causing excruciating pain all around my shoulder area. Walking was difficult for a while however I was determined to visit Lorraine as I had heard great reports about how well she looked already. When I got the strength on that second day I went to see her. What a transformation in her whole appearance. Before her face had been almost yellow and her eyes very sunk into her face. Already I could see such a change. Her eyes were shining and her skin colour already changed. It was a miracle! What a reward, to see such a change so quickly. Lorraine couldn't say the same for me. She still reminds me at times how poorly I looked, gasping for breath with each step and unable to straighten. She was so concerned for me but with each passing day my recovery was swift and by the fifth day I was ready for home.

Family visited us both while we were in hospital. My mum and dad came together. My sister and her daughter Rebecca arrived and Eleanor my sister said a lovely prayer over me. My daughter Jaclyn arrived during the third day bringing me popcorn, my weakness! It was Lorraine's dads visit that was particularly special. Ben had already lost his wife to the same disease and never liked hospitals much. However nothing was going to stop him from coming to see how Lorraine looked. After seeing her he came into visit me. Tears were in his eyes as he thanked me. We hugged and I just knew how much God loved him too and at that moment I understood this was all for him too.

Surgery had all gone successfully. Doctors were all on standby on the third day, which can be the crucial day for rejection to show up. However it didn't. Lorraine even asked for chips to be brought in from the local chip shop, something she hadn't been able to enjoy with salt for so long! The kidney itself must have been a perfect specimen because Lorraine was wheeled down for a scan one morning and got quite alarmed, wondering was something wrong. However the doctor explained that because the kidney was so perfect and surgery had gone perfectly too they wanted the young doctors to see how this looked.

Every test carried out was another test passed. Nothing went wrong after surgery. Even the doctors were amazed. I headed home first and by the end of the week Lorraine was able to keep her promise to Madge and arrived home on time! What a day of celebration.

In the weeks which followed we both had check ups. Mine was only one trip to check my wound. Lorraine had twice weekly trips, which eventually dropped to fortnightly and today two and half years on, she only attends once every three months.

To call this a success story, really doesn't do it justice. It was truly a miracle of God. The smoothness of pre surgery and post surgery left us both rendered speechless. What a great God. That's what he is capable of you see. He takes a broken vessel moulds it, reshapes it and fashions it into something new. I was that old broken vessel. I m very happy with his workmanship.

Many months after the surgery Lorraine and I were asked to go and tell our story to my local church in Ballymena called Dwelling Place. Pastor Eugene allowed us the evening service to tell of Gods wonderful act of healing. All my close family attended to hear my testimony, along with Lorraine's. It was such an opportunity to give all the glory back to God. It was a beautiful conclusion to share our story with people who had been so faithful in praying for us during that whole period. Many wanted to see for themselves what God had done.

Following that meeting we were asked to speak at many more fellowships, all wanting to hear what God had done. So you see the surgery brought so much more. Not only did Lorraine get her life back but it gave us such a wonderful story to go tell of his glory. This story was never going to be about me but all about him. Without him it would never have happened. He was the master planner. When he knit me in my mothers womb, one of my kidneys had Lorraine's name on it! He made a way when there was no way. He brought hope to Lorraine when there was no hope. He took her illness and cancelled it. He took all the heavy chains off all her family members and gave them back their freedom from years of dialysis at home. He gave me a story. He platformed my life to give him all the glory and that's all I want to do. I truly believe as I end this book that my God has a spare kidney in heaven which he can supernaturally transplant into my body. There is nothing too great for my God. So as I finish I'm aware there is another chapter still to conclude.He is asking me to exercise my faith and believe for supernatural transplant. Will you dear reader walk with me believing for this?

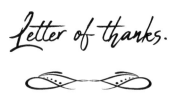

Letter of thanks.

*M*any church groups in our home town of larne and surrounding villages had began to hear about our imminent surgery and were praying about it. We wish to say thank you to all those men and women who took time to remember us in this way. We mention those we know of. Ladies meeting in Straid, Broughshane, Ballyclare, Cairncastle, and Ballymena. To all those groups we want to say a huge thank you. To know that we had so many praying for us over that period, really held us up and kept us strong. As we travel around we continue to meet people who say they were praying for us. That is so humbling that just by word of mouth, you took time to think of us. We continue to remain so thankful to our God for his lovely miracle of healing and if this book has encouraged anyone in their faith then it has been a success. It was never meant to be about us but all about our loving saviour. We give him all the thanks and glory

Lightning Source UK Ltd.
Milton Keynes UK
UKHW022215200619
344748UK00007B/262/P